AN INTRODUCTION
TO HUMAN BLOOD GROUPS

AN INTRODUCTION
TO
HUMAN BLOOD GROUPS

by

FULTON ROBERTS, M.D.

Fellow of Jesus College, Cambridge, and
Lecturer in Pathology in the Univerity.

1960

WILLIAM HEINEMANN · MEDICAL BOOKS · LTD

LONDON

First published 1960

PRINTED IN GREAT BRITAIN BY THE WHITEFRIARS PRESS LTD.
LONDON AND TONBRIDGE

CONTENTS

The Peripatetic's Problem

"Send at once to the operating-theatre two units of freshly drawn ACD blood." I debated with myself, does this mean Group A, type Rh_1 blood, or blood freshly drawn into acid-citrate-dextrose solution? In view of the emergency I decided to send group O, Rh-negative blood, which I duly marked with its blood type O dd. A few minutes later the telephone rang. "What's wrong with this blood? It looks all right to us." I replied, "There is nothing wrong with the blood." "Then why have you marked 'Odd' blood all over the place?"

I am indebted to the editor of The Lancet *for permission to quote a peripatetic correspondent; and to Blackwell Scientific Publications (Oxford) for permission to quote from Race and Sanger's "Blood Groups in Man."*

PREFACE

THE publication of *The Rhesus Factor* in 1947 was intended to assist those who at that time found the topic bewildering. The ensuing decade has not only rendered that book out of perspective but also provided many other succinct expositions of the subject for the reader's use. It may be, however, that the rapid rate of increase in knowledge that twelve years ago caused the Rh blood groups to appear confusing, is today engendering a similar perplexity concerning human blood groups as a whole. To those who find it so this work is offered as a simple introduction to the topic in the hope that it may be found useful.

In 1949 I was taken to task by a reviewer for pretending that the rhesus factor was indeed a difficult subject. " His only armour is an algebraic nomenclature, stripped of which he stands revealed as the mere clinical application of a very simple principle of immunity. . . . Nevertheless there is a strong rumour abroad that the Rh factor is hopelessly complicated, capable of analysis only by the most acute . . . it would be so much better to let the doctor straightway into the secret . . . that certain clinical facts have been obscured by much published laboratory data. It is quite an ordinary message, but it has been ciphered by those serologists with their cabbalistic signs and hieroglyphs." I range myself on the side of the reviewer, departing from his view only in ascribing the " cabbalistic signs and hieroglyphs " as much to geneticists as to serologists. It is the notation of blood groups, including the Rh groups, that is a prime source of confusion and this is very much a genetical matter. The reader of this book may feel that the time for a revision of blood-group notation is near, and that it will justify the temporary inconvenience of being obliged to become adapted to a new system.

The immunological features of blood groups are quite straightforward and differ little from those of bacteriology. As it is this aspect of the topic that will principally concern the clinician I have ventured to introduce this account with a chapter on elementary serological matters.

There is, however, one other potential source of difficulty that I have sought to remove. It is common practice for the student to enter the topic of blood groups by a consideration first of the ABO system. This is no doubt partly because of its cardinal clinical importance and its priority in discovery. But this practice implies that the ABO system is both simple and typical, a view which I do not share. The order in which I have presented the material, and which I believe to be logical, leaves the ABO system almost till the last. The reader who wishes to learn only about the Rhesus factor (D) and the ABO system can omit Chapters V to VII without impairing the continuity of the account. An objection may be raised against my order, namely that the reader must carry in his mind the presumption of ABO compatibility throughout all the earlier chapters which deal with the other groups ; but this need applies to the bench alone.

No citation of authorities is given in the text, but a short bibliography has been compiled at the end. Needless to say the chief source to which the interested reader will wish to turn for further detail is Race and Sanger's splendid book *Blood Groups in Man*, from which, with the consent of authors and publishers, I have quoted a figure and relevant text on p. 53. I am most grateful to Dr. Race for reading this manuscript before publication.

CAMBRIDGE, G. F. R.
August 1959.

CHAPTER I

SEROLOGICAL INTRODUCTION

If the blood of a certain animal—say the sheep—is introduced into an animal of a different species—say the rabbit—one of the consequences will be the appearance of antibodies in the serum of the recipient. The most important property of these antibodies is that they will combine with and react with samples of the injected material, or material containing the same chemical substances; and this process of combination and reaction may be observed either *in vivo* or *in vitro*.

Antibody formation is brought about by the parenteral access of foreign material—that is to say, material which does not form any part of the recipient's organism. Thus no animal normally forms antibodies against any substance that is part of itself or of its biological inheritance. Not all foreign material will evoke antibodies in the recipient, but nearly all proteins of substantial molecular weight will do so, and there are a few non-protein substances that have this power. Often the foreign molecule contains protein but the antibody shows a disposition to combine particularly with the non-protein parts of it. Such antibody-provoking substances are called antigens. The antibodies that arise are serum globulins moving with the gamma fraction.

On the first occasion that a subject encounters a foreign substance the response is relatively slow. The antibody-producing cells, whichever these may be, do not provide a rapid accumulation of antibody and it may be a fortnight or more before there is provided an excess of antibody sufficient, after union with the injected antigen, to be detectable in the free state in the recipient's serum. The quantity of antibody in the serum then rises very slowly to a maximum by about six weeks after the injection, and thereafter steadily declines.

On the second, and subsequent occasions, however, the response is more rapid and antibody may flood the circulation seven to ten days after exposure to the antigen. Once the subject has made antibody against a certain antigen he may be described as "immunised" to this antigen and remains in that state for life, so far as can be judged. This must not be taken to imply that there are always antibodies present in the immunised subject's serum throughout life, far from it. But once immunised, the rapid antibody response (called the secondary immune response) will always follow any exposure to the antigen however long this may be after the first encounter. It follows that the amount of antibody detectable in a patient's serum is no index of the degree of immunity and is of limited practical value as an isolated observation.

Another important property of antibodies is their specificity. Each chemical substance in the injected material provokes its own antibody that will unite with it and act independently of the others. In the example mentioned, of injecting sheep's blood into a rabbit, the recipient would form antibodies against substances found in the serum of the sheep as well as those on the red cells of the sheep. If the sheep cells had been washed free of serum before injection, only antibodies against the red cells would be provoked in the rabbit. And as sheep red cells have a number of chemically distinct antigens on their surface, so several independent antibodies would be formed in consequence.

The presence of such antibodies in the recipient's serum may normally be recognised *in vitro* by two common laboratory reactions. The first of these would be by showing the power of the antibody to lyse the appropriate red cells in the presence of fresh guinea-pig serum as a source of complement, the whole test being conducted at body temperature. This procedure (immune hæmolysis) is rarely adopted in routine work on human blood groups ; it is mentioned again in only one context in Chapter VIII. But it is worth remembering that this is very probably what happens *in vivo* when blood is injected into an animal that has already formed antibodies against the injected cells ; the existing antibody and the ever-present complement cause the cells to break down, and the danger to the recipient results from the difficulty in disposing of these damaged cells.

The other method of recognising antibodies against red cells is by agglutination. Antibodies against red cells will, in most cases, cause cells of chemical constitution similar to those that provoked the formation of the antibody to agglutinate, that is, to adhere together in large clumps. Not all antibodies against red cells can cause agglutination and these exceptions are considered in Chapter IV in some detail.

The normal way of estimating by agglutination the quantity of antibody in the serum of an immunised animal is to prepare a series of increasing dilutions of the serum being studied, to which are added equal volumes of a suspension of red cells of appropriate antigenic constitution. The greatest dilution that effects agglutination is noted (say, 200 times, or a dilution of 1 in 200) and this is called the titre ; it would usually be expressed as " 200 " in the example given. This is not, of course, an absolute measure, nor is it particularly accurate. But it serves as a comparison of the amounts of antibody in the serum of different animals, or of the same animal at different times.

It may be necessary to identify and separate several

antibodies in one serum. To reconsider the original example of injecting sheep cells into a rabbit, suppose the sheep's cell contained two antigens, S found only in the sheep and G found also in goats. If the serum is tested against sheep cells and goat cells the titre might be the same in each case, say 200.

To differentiate between the two antibodies it would be necessary to " absorb " the serum successively with sheep cells and goat cells. Absorption consists of exposing a portion of serum to an excess of cells for a period of time to permit union of antibody with antigen. The sample is then spun in a centrifuge and the serum decanted and the cells discarded. When this process has been repeated two or three times with fresh cells it can be assumed that all the antibody against those cells has been removed from the serum. In the example the result might be as in the Table I.

TABLE I

Absorption	Tested against	Titre
None	Sheep cells	200
	Goat cells	200
With sheep cells	Sheep cells	nil
	Goat cells	nil
With goat cells	Sheep cells	50
	Goat cells	nil

The serum thus contains anti-G in a titre of 200 and anti-S in a titre of 50.

The example mentioned—the injection of sheep cells into a rabbit—illustrates another matter. Most rabbits already contain in their serum antibodies that agglutinate sheep cells, though it cannot be supposed that they have in fact encountered sheep cells at any time. These are called "naturally-occurring" antibodies, implying that they are not known certainly to result from exposure to the antigen concerned. There are no doubt many objections to referring to them thus, for they may not be naturally-occurring and are not typical as antibodies, but as they are frequently encountered in blood-group work it is desirable to be able to refer to them until a fuller understanding enables us to label them more precisely.

The immunisation of one species with washed red cells from another is an example of *hetero-immunisation*. One might enquire what happens if blood from one member of a species is injected into another member of the same species. If red blood cells in all members of a given species were identical in chemical composition no antibodies would be evolved. In fact, however, the red cells of some members of a species differ chemically from those of other members of that species, and these differences, which are inherited, are called blood groups. This is as true of the horse, cow, sheep and rabbit as it is of man, but only human blood groups are to be considered here. The injection of blood from one member of the human species into another, as happens quite commonly now that blood transfusion is widespread, may result in antibody formation if certain precautions are omitted ; this may be called *iso-immunisation*. Iso-immunisation in man is attended by certain dangers to health ; it also provides the antibodies by means of which human blood groups are studied. It is of these matters that this book treats.

CHAPTER II

THE RHESUS FACTOR

THE discovery of the ABO groups by Landsteiner in 1900 was the first demonstration of human blood groups. They did not assume clinical importance until the discovery of citrate as a harmless anticoagulant rendered blood transfusion a practicable procedure about the time of the First World War. And it was not until the Second World War that transfusion became so widespread a practice that a knowledge of blood groups became an indispensable part of the pathologist's equipment. Blood groups other than ABO had been discovered in 1927 (M, N and P, also by Landsteiner associated with Levine) but they evoked little interest as they were of no clinical importance. On the other hand the discovery of the Rhesus factor in 1940 (also by Landsteiner associated with Wiener) aroused very considerable and widespread interest. There were three reasons for this ; first, it was clearly demonstrated that this new blood group could cause disease among infants as well as being responsible for transfusion reactions ; secondly, the considerable increase in transfusions in the early days of the war brought these dangers into prominence, and, thirdly, the interesting properties of the Rhesus factor gave new stimulus to the several fields of study associated with blood groups, namely serology, genetics and anthropology.

The Rhesus factor was discovered during the course of some experiments in which blood of the Rhesus monkey (*Macacus rhesus*) was being injected into rabbits. The sera of the rabbits agglutinated all samples of the monkey cells, as would be expected, but they also agglutinated some, but not all, of the samples of human red cells to which they were exposed. This observation implied that some, but not all, individuals of the human species had a red-cell antigen that was universal among rhesus monkeys. The proportion of people possessing the monkey's antigen among those sampled in New York was about 85 per cent. and a similar incidence was found in Britain ; this varies considerably, however, in different parts of the world and among other races. The antigen thus became known as the Rhesus factor, and those possessing it were termed "Rhesus positive" and those lacking it were "Rhesus negative." The latter terms, which are still in use, are generally abbreviated to Rh positive and Rh negative. The antigen is no longer called the Rh factor, for reasons that will appear later, and is now referred to as the blood-group antigen D. The distribution of D is quite independent of A, B and O.

Rh positive persons, therefore, carry the antigen D on their red cells. Rh negative persons lack this antigen but may be regarded as possessing instead an antigen called d.* These substances are inherited according to mendelian law and it is likely that there are genes for D and d, one or other of which occupies a certain site on the chromosome. The several genes of which one will occupy a certain site on the chromosome are called alleles. Each individual receives paired chromosomes, one from each parent, so that a rhesus negative person will have received two d's and his genotype will be expressed as dd. Rhesus positive persons may have received two D's, having thus a genotype of DD ; but they may alternatively have received one of each type, so that their genotype would be Dd. In the former case the state is referred to as homo-

* As a matter of fact the existence of d is not proved, nor that of the antibody, anti-d ; but the present argument may be allowed to stand until p. 35.

zygous and in the latter heterozygous ; rhesus negative persons, of course, are all homozygous.

TABLE II

	Genotypes	
Rhesus positive	DD	(homozygous)
	or Dd	(heterozygous)
Rhesus negative	dd	(homozygous)

A word on the use of certain symbols might be convenient at this point. The letters D and d may refer, according to the context, either to the genes themselves or to the antigens on the red cell resulting from the action of these genes. In practice it is nearly always apparent which construction is to be placed on the symbols, but it has been recommended that the distinction should be made by using italics thus, *DD*, when genes are being referred to and leaving the roman type to express antigens. It has not been thought necessary to adopt this practice here but it will doubtless become increasingly employed with benefit to clarity.

Another source of confusion is the adoption of capital and small letters to distinguish between those two alleles. This practice may give rise to the erroneous impression that D is a mendelian dominant and d a recessive character. This is not true. The difference between a dominant and recessive character is that the recessive cannot be recognised if the dominant is present in the same individual. If an anti-d antibody* were produced in a DD person by injection of dd cells, and could be shown to agglutinate Dd cells, then d would be as dominant as D. In practice both D and d are regarded as of equal dominance.

It is true that it is much easier to produce anti-D in an Rh

* See note on p. 15.

negative person than anti-d in an Rh positive one, but this is because D is a very powerful antigen and d an exceptionally weak one. The difference between D and d, therefore, is not at a genetic level but an antigenic one ; the whole importance of D, the Rhesus factor, is solely due to its being a very powerful antigen.

Its importance has become particularly emphasised by the considerable increase in the use of blood transfusion during the last twenty years. About one white person in seven is rhesus negative and if blood were administered regardless of Rh grouping the chances of such a person receiving rhesus positive blood would be about 6 to 1. As about half the number of rhesus negative people so transfused (for the first time) would produce antibody it can be calculated that random transfusion regardless of Rh group would produce anti-D antibodies in about one in every sixteen persons transfused.

It may be thought that to cause a patient to produce Rh antibodies in his serum is not particularly serious, for no ill-effects follow and patient and doctor alike may be unaware that immunisation has occurred. It is true that on the first occasion of this happening no detectable damage may result. But should the patient require a subsequent transfusion a severe reaction is almost certain to follow the administration of D positive blood.

Transfusion reactions result from administering to a patient blood containing an antigen against which there is already an antibody present in the patient's circulation. The antibody causes the destruction of the transfused cells. In mild cases this may take no more serious a form than an increased rate of elimination of the transfused cells from the recipient's circulation, and the worst that can be said is that the transfusion can have done no good. In more severe cases, however, the rapid destruction of the cells causes the symptoms of a transfusion reaction, sweating, pain in the loins, restlessness and, in severe cases, partial or complete suppression of urine. The principal danger to the patient is the damage to the kidneys that may result from the rapid destruction of the transfused red cells by the patient's antibody. Consideration will later be given to the steps necessary to ensure that the donor's and recipient's blood are compatible.

CHAPTER III

HÆMOLYTIC DISEASE OF THE NEWBORN

THE discovery of the Rhesus factor in 1940 was opportune. During the previous decade the number of transfusion reactions when the ABO groups were known to be compatible was exciting comment. And at the same time explanations were being advanced for certain disorders of newborn children occurring in several members of the same family, that were based on a supposed incompatibility between mother and child. It was thus soon apparent that the Rhesus factor was responsible for both these anomalies. The transfusion reactions were shown to be due to incompatibility of the Rh blood groups and brought about by anti-D. And the mothers of the sick children were also shown to have Rh antibodies in their serum which had damaged the red cells of their fœtuses, giving rise to a condition called hæmolytic disease of the newborn.

What was not clear was how these maternal antibodies had arisen. Undoubtedly in a number of cases the antibodies had been evoked by incompatible transfusion. In others, however, no evidence could be obtained of any transfusions having been administered to the mothers at any time, and anti-D has never been shown to occur naturally. There was considerable speculation about whether the fœtus itself could provoke antibody production in the mother. It is true that the fœtus could be Rh positive even in a rhesus negative mother, the positivity (D) being inherited from the father ; but it was not easy to see how the fœtal blood could pass from child to mother to provoke antibody formation in the latter, the placenta seeming to present a barrier impassable by red cells.

Recently it has been shown, however, that it is quite possible for fœtal blood to enter the maternal veins. In some circumstances a hæmorrhage of unknown cause may arise from the fœtal side of the placenta so that at parturition, or even before, some of this blood may enter the dilated uterine sinuses of the mother. This being so, one would not expect any firstborn child to suffer from this condition, for the mother would not become immunised until her first parturition was accomplished. This is indeed true and, with very rare exceptions, no first-born child is affected with the disease unless, of course, the mother had already been immunised by incompatible blood transfusion.

To sum up, therefore, one can say that only rhesus negative mothers are vulnerable, and only those married to rhesus positive fathers can bear vulnerable infants. The rhesus negative mothers may have been immunised against D by incompatible transfusion and, if so, all their rhesus positive children would be exposed to the antibody. If these immunised mothers were married to homozygous (DD) husbands, all their children would be rhesus positive and at risk, for DD $\times$ dd can give rise only to Dd. But those married to heterozygous (Dd) husbands could bear some rhesus negative offspring (Dd $\times$ dd $=$ Dd *or* dd) who would not be threatened, for dd infants would be unaffected by an anti-D antibody.

It follows from these considerations that the transfusion of Rh positive blood into an Rh negative female before or during the child-bearing period of life is an error of such gravity that it may deprive her of the opportunity of ever bearing a live child. No single fact in the whole realm of blood-group study is more important than this. If, however, it is made the rule never to transfuse any female that has not passed the menopause without first determining her blood group, and to administer only rhesus negative blood to those who prove to be rhesus negative, then no woman will be artificially immunised against D. And if this is so, then the incidence of hæmolytic disease due to the antigen D will be no greater than the incidence of retro-placental hæmorrhage in rhesus negative mothers. Not only is this incidence low, but such mothers as are immunised in this way may expect at least one child, their first, to be unaffected by the disease. It is important to emphasise that the natural incidence of the condition is very low, and though about one marriage in ten is between a rhesus negative wife and a rhesus positive husband, only in about one in twenty of such marriages is there any evidence of hæmolytic disease ; and in most of these the disease is mild and in many of the others it can be successfully treated.

The cause of the disease, as has been explained, is the immunisation of rhesus negative mothers against the Rh antigen D. But it is the children, not the mothers, who suffer from hæmolytic disease. The mother's antibody, anti-D, can reach the fœtus *in utero* as nearly all antibodies can, probably by passing directly across the placenta though other routes have been suggested. The infant's circulation can thus be flooded with anti-D during pregnancy so that the red cells of Rh positive infants will be subjected to a continuing and destructive bombardment with the maternal antibody.

Very little is known about how the fœtus disposes of the broken-down red cells and their products *in utero*, but one would suppose that anæmia would invariably be a consequence of these circumstances, and so it is. In very mild cases there may be no other abnormality, and the fœtus, having adapted itself successfully to its anoxic environment *in utero*, is born with a mild anæmia which may pass undetected: a condition formerly known as *congenital anæmia of the newborn.* It is, however, slow to mend and the bone marrow responds very sluggishly during the first few weeks of life when, in any case, there is also a heavy demand for red cells because of the growth in size, and hence of circulatory volume, of the newborn infant. Thus the danger in these cases, which are not common, is that the neonatal anæmia is overlooked and the child is found *in extremis* two or three weeks later.

At the other end of the scale, in the very severe cases the antibody exerts such widespread damage on the red cells *in utero* that the fœtus succumbs before birth. The effect of such extreme anæmia *in utero* is to disturb, in some way, the fluid balance of the fœtus with the result that there is generalised œdema. The condition is thus known as *hydrops fœtalis.* It is not common but it is fatal, for even the few infants born alive succumb within a few hours, or at most, a day.

The most common manifestation of this disease, however, lies between these two extremes and differs from each. The infant is born, often prematurely, with some degree of anæmia and with a considerable amount of maternal antibody still in its circulation. Once this antibody is excreted, as like most foreign substances it will be, there is no further cause for deterioration. But in the neonatal period the antibody will continue to destroy red cells probably as fast as the bone marrow (and other centres) can make them. So the anæmia rapidly worsens and may kill the child.

Fortunately infants with this condition do not seem to suffer any renal disorder in consequence of trying to dispose of broken-down red cells as would an adult receiving an incompatible blood transfusion. But the infant does have difficulty in disposing of one product of excessive red-cell destruction, namely, bilirubin. How the fœtus disposes of excess bilirubin *in utero* is not clear, but it certainly succeeds in doing so. After birth, however, the excessive rate of red-cell destruction liberates more bilirubin than the neonatal liver can handle so that bilirubin accumulates in the circulation and the infant soon becomes deeply jaundiced. Jaundice being so prominent a feature of the condition, it is called *icterus gravis neonatorum*, and is the third of the syndromes that make up hæmolytic disease of the newborn.

A word about bilirubin may be helpful at this point. The bilirubin that is formed from the breakdown of hæmoglobin is recognised by the indirect van den Bergh reaction. It passes in the circulation to the liver where it is conjugated with glucuronic acid and secreted into the bile. The conjugated form is recognised by the direct van den Bergh reaction, and it differs from the unconjugated form in being more soluble. The clinical differences between the hæmolytic and obstructive types of jaundice illustrate the chemical differences between the two forms of bilirubin. It has been suggested that the name "bilirubin" be reserved to the product of hæmoglobin breakdown before it reaches the liver, and that the conjugated form be distinguished by being called simply "conjugated bilirubin." In hæmolytic disease it is bilirubin proper, and not the conjugated form, that is concerned.

The jaundice in hæmolytic disease exposes the infant to another peril. It seems that during the first week of life the endothelium of the vessels in the brain have not yet acquired the impermeability that later protects brain tissue from certain substances that might damage it and which may be found in the circulation. Bilirubin is one of these, and there is no evidence that in normal circumstances bilirubin ever reaches the brain in adult jaundice of any form. But in infancy the bilirubin not only reaches the brain but, once there, interferes with the tissue oxidation of certain cells, particularly those of the basal ganglia, and also stains them. This may happen in other parts of the body, but certain brain cells seem to be particularly vulnerable and many of them die. The result is a serious neurological disturbance in the first week of life, called *kernicterus*, which frequently kills the infants or leaves signs of permanent residual damage of the brain in those that survive.

It might be thought that kernicterus would develop from other causes of jaundice in the first week of life. It does not do so in congenital obliteration of the bile duct, partly because jaundice may arise later than the first week, and perhaps because the conjugated form of bilirubin, which is here concerned, may be less toxic for brain tissue. Kernicterus may develop, however, in premature infants, particularly those that have received large doses of vitamin K. In these premature infants the liver is not yet fully developed and takes some time to mature. Hence several days may elapse after birth before the liver can conjugate bilirubin at the rate required even for normal red-cell breakdown and the pigment accumulates in the blood. Administration of excessive vitamin K worsens the situation by promoting some hæmolysis of the infant's cells.

The infant with hæmolytic disease is thus threatened with two dangers. The first of these is anæmia, mild in the case of congenital anæmia : so severe as to be irremediably fatal in hydrops fœtalis : and of considerable and worsening severity in icterus gravis. The second danger is that of kernicterus following an accumulation of bilirubin during the first week of life. The severity of these two processes is to some extent independent of each other for, though the increased blood destruction causes anæmia and predisposes to kernicterus, it is the degree of immaturity of the liver that finally determines the severity of the latter.

Many of the signs and symptoms of hæmolytic disease of the newborn have been referred to in discussing the natural history of the disease, but there are others that merit mention. In all forms of the disease, other than the mildest anæmias, the liver and spleen are enlarged, indicating a prolongation into extra-uterine life of the use of tissue in these organs for erythropoietic purposes. There is also a bleeding tendency, which can be marked ; indeed, in the nineteenth century so many infants with this disorder died of umbilical hæmorrhage that it was thought that such hæmorrhage might be a hereditary characteristic so often did it exhibit itself in families. In severe cases the signs of anæmic heart failure with raised venous pressure may be found. In all cases there is lethargy and difficulty with feeding, and all the symptoms and signs, which are manifest very quickly after birth, reach their height between the third and eighth days. Finally there is an element of apparent toxicity in all but the mildest cases, most noticeable when kernicterus is super-imposed. Kernicterus itself is principally characterised by local or general hypertonicity often spasmodic, deafness and, terminally, pulmonary hæmorrhages.

It has already been mentioned that the firstborn infant usually escapes hæmolytic disease, and an explanation of this fact has been offered. What has not been explicitly stated is a much less easily explained fact that once a mother has become immunised against the D antigen and borne an affected child, all her subsequent Rh positive children are also affected. This is an important fact, for though immunisation is uncommon, once it occurs the problem is serious, particularly, of course, in families whose firstborn is sick or dead from other causes. It is important to determine if the father is homozygous or heterozygous, for if he is the latter (D/d) some rhesus negative, and therefore unaffected, children can be expected.

It is not easy to explain this continuing morbidity from a single cause in one family. It might be that the initial immunisation could provoke enough antibody to kill or harm successive Rh positive infants over a period of five or ten years ; but there is as yet insufficient evidence on this point. If, on the other hand, a new antigenic stimulus arises with each pregnancy it is difficult to see why retro-placental hæmorrhage from the fœtus should occur invariably with some mothers and never with others. This matter is not well understood and some light might be thrown on the matter if it could be shown that the disease in the subsequent children was regularly more severe, or less severe, or regularly increased or decreased in severity. There is no absolute rule about this and, indeed, the prompt application of treatment hinders uncomplicated assessment of this matter. But there is a general impression that in some families the disease on the whole continues to be mild in all the siblings, whereas in others the disease remains severe or worsens. This observation may not help in determining the cause of the condition, but is important in considering the advice to offer to a family about prognosis and treatment.

There are three forms of treatment which need to be considered. The first is that which applies only to those infants that are discovered to have a severe anæmia in the second or third week of life ; they need a transfusion of rhesus negative blood. The second and most important form of treatment is exchange transfusion which is applied soon after birth. In this a plastic catheter is passed up the umbilical vein into the vena cava and a 20 ml. syringe with a three-way tap is attached. This allows an alternating withdrawal, discarding and replacement of 20 ml. volumes of blood. The blood used for replacement should be rhesus negative (so that it is unaffected by the antibody) fresh (to ameliorate the bleeding tendency) and partly packed (to provide good oxygen-carrying power without overloading the circulation).

This procedure enables a number of the infant's ills to be corrected. In the first place rather more blood can be withdrawn than is replaced, which relieves the raised venous pressure that may accompany anæmic heart failure. Secondly the discarding of the infant's own blood disposes not only of the antibody that is destroying its cells but also some of the bilirubin that is damaging its brain. Finally the provision of rhesus negative cells tides the infant over the dangerous neonatal period of anæmia until the antibody is finally excreted and a new population of its own rhesus positive cells has arisen. Properly applied exchange transfusion is safe and curative. It underlines the need for ante-natal diagnosis so that delivery in hospital, where proper facilities are available, can be ensured. Hence every pregnant mother must be rhesus grouped, and antibodies sought towards the end of pregnancy in those that are rhesus negative. If this were regularly done it would enable all those that might require hospital treatment to be admitted, and greatly reduce the mortality from this disease. This extremely important point should not be overlooked, for this is one of the occasions, rare in medical practice, when disease can be anticipated by preparedness.

The indications for exchange transfusion can be easily assessed. The infant is threatened with two possible causes of death, anæmia or kernicterus, each of which needs consideration in the individual case. The risk from anæmia can usually be gauged from the cord hæmoglobin level. If this is less than 15 G per 100 ml. it is wise to transfuse, for experience has taught that in these cases the level soon falls quite abruptly. The cord bilirubin level is not, however, any guide to the risk of kernicterus, for it cannot be a measure of post-natal liver function. The serum bilirubin level must, therefore, be estimated periodically during the first two days of life (or longer in some cases), and exchange transfusion is called for if a level of 20 mgm. per 100 ml. is exceeded.

There has been considerable debate for some time about the value of the third form of treatment, premature induction of labour. There are sound reasons for believing that in the majority of cases the infant is probably better adapted *in utero* to anoxia and to bilirubin excess than it would be post-natally, when its liver would be very immature and its general health prejudiced by the consequences of prematurity. There is much to be said, therefore, for allowing the pregnancy to go to term in the hope, among other things, that the liver will be relatively mature. Nevertheless, there are undoubtedly cases that benefit from early induction of labour. By way of example, perhaps a little exaggerated, one may consider the position of a mother who has lost her first child from pneumonia and the next three, stillborn, from hydrops fœtalis. The outlook in such a case, if the father is homozygous, is extremely unfavourable and it is to be doubted whether, without assistance, such a mother could ever expect to bear a living child. With such a prognosis, early induction, followed by exchange transfusion, probably repeated several times, offers the best hope of saving the child. It has also been suggested that the mother's antibody titre should be under continuous observation during pregnancy so that labour could be induced at once if the titre suddenly rises in the last few weeks before term.

Hæmolytic disease may also arise, though not commonly, from immunisation against blood groups other than D, when it takes much the same course as is here described. But one important and not uncommon exception is when the A and B groups are responsible for the disease, a matter discussed on page 59.

CHAPTER IV

RHESUS ANTIBODIES

THE rhesus antibody (anti-D), discovered in 1940, displays two properties that might go some way towards explaining why it was not detected earlier. First, the agglutinated clumps of cells are sometimes loosely held together, and are easily dispersed on shaking. Secondly, anti-D agglutinates effectively only at body temperature. The somewhat crude blood-grouping techniques that had been considered adequate hitherto (*e.g.* shaking antiserum and cells together on a tile at room temperature) would not have revealed the action of anti-D at all easily.

A further reason why anti-D must commonly have gone unrecognised was revealed by some most important observations made in 1944, namely that some samples of anti-D could be shown to have united with the red cells without having agglutinated them. Of course, there are circumstances in which such a state of affairs is not at all remarkable. For example (as has already been described) an antibody against sheep cells prepared in the rabbit might agglutinate the appropriate cells when it was diluted 200 times but not when diluted 2,000 times ; nevertheless, in the latter case some antibody can be shown to be attached to the cells, for the addition of some guinea-pig complement would effect lysis of the cells. The difference here is quantitative ; but this is not the explanation of the failure of some samples of anti-D to bring about agglutination, for they fail whatever their strength.

Normally the agglutination reaction is divided arbitrarily into two stages. In the first stage antibody becomes attached to (sensitises) the cells, and in the second stage the cells come together in clumps. Evidently some samples of anti-D could effect only the first stage and hence they were called "incomplete" antibodies to distinguish them from the agglutinating samples of anti-D. Since practically all blood-group work from 1900 until 1944 had been based on the agglutination reaction, it is easy to see that these incomplete antibodies would not have been detected.

Incomplete anti-D does not differ from agglutinating anti-D in specificity: each reacts only with cells containing D. If both forms of antibody are present in the same serum it is usually the incomplete form that succeeds in uniting with the antigen on the cell surface, often to the exclusion of the agglutinating form. Cells sensitised in this way by incomplete anti-D would not be agglutinated by agglutinating anti-D because their D antigens would already be occupied ("blocked" in serological jargon). There are grounds for believing that the incomplete form reaches the fœtus more easily and is therefore more dangerous in hæmolytic disease of the newborn.

A number of methods for detecting incomplete anti-D have been developed of which three (and their variants) are in general use. The first of these is to employ certain diluents other than saline as a suspending medium. The use of human plasma or 20 per cent. bovine albumin or dextran of suitable strength as a testing medium usually enables incomplete anti-D to agglutinate Rh positive cells. The albumin test is very convenient in routine blood-group work and is, on the whole, reliable, but some samples of incomplete anti-D will be missed by this method.

The second technique, which is also quite simple and useful, is to treat the cells under standard conditions with dilute solutions of certain proteolytic enzymes of which trypsin, ficin and papain are known to be effective. This treatment renders Rh positive cells agglutinable by nearly all samples of incomplete anti-D. This is a reliable test in skilled hands, but there is always the risk that over-treatment of the cells may result in panagglutinability.

The third technique is the antiglobulin reaction or Coombs test. Rhesus positive red cells carry a number of D antigens scattered over their surface to which the incomplete anti-D antibodies become attached. Since these antibodies are composed (as all antibodies are) of serum globulin, one can picture the sensitised red cell as having human globulin likewise scattered over the surface in the distribution of the D antigen. An antibody against human globulin would thus cause these cells to agglutinate. An antibody can easily be prepared against human globulin by injecting this substance in any animal that is not human. In practice human serum is injected into rabbits or goats, and the resulting antiserum, after being absorbed with human cells, will agglutinate only those cells that have incomplete antibody absorbed on their surface, *i.e.* sensitised cells.

The test is, therefore, very usefully applied to newborn infant's cells ; if it is positive, the cells are sensitised and the only source of antibody is the mother, hence a diagnosis of hæmolytic disease can be made with certainty. Likewise, a negative test would exclude the disease (but see p. 60). It is the most valuable single test in the diagnosis of hæmolytic disease. It is also useful in detecting incomplete antibody in serum, by exposing Rh positive cells to the serum and, after washing the cells, testing them with an antiglobulin serum. The cells need to be washed thoroughly whenever the test is performed, for any human serum not attached to the cells would neutralise the antiglobulin serum before it could agglutinate the cells. This test is reliable for all blood group systems, but the trypsin and albumin tests, though useful for anti-D, fail to react in some systems.

These three tests are all in use in routine blood-group work and enable the incomplete antibody to be detected and measured as accurately as the agglutinating form. Titrations of anti-D however, are of only moderate value for clinical assessment, both because techniques differ among laboratories and also because the severity of the infant's illness is by no means always correlated with the maternal antibody titre. But it has been claimed that continuous observation of the mother's level of antibody, determined by the antiglobulin test, would enable the clinician to detect promptly any marked change that might adversely affect the fœtus and to reconsider the possible forms of treatment.

Perhaps the most important consideration about anti-D from the point of view of clinical practice is its scarcity. Rh grouping can be carried out only by the use of anti-D, agglutinating or incomplete. The only source of anti-D is the immunised patient. The prevention of disease due to anti-D can therefore be fostered best by arranging that those immunised patients who can spare a little blood at the appropriate time should be bled by the Regional Transfusion Service and their serum made available. Twenty ml. of serum would suffice for several hundred tests.

CHAPTER V

THE Rh COMPLEX

VERY soon after the discovery of D and anti-D it became clear from independent work in Britain and America that other closely related but distinct reactions were regularly observable. Some additional antigens with their respective antibodies were evidently closely associated with the Rh antigen D. It is possible to construct a table to show the relationship between the four antibodies that had been studied by the end of 1943 (Table III).

TABLE III

Antibody No. 1	+	−	−	−	−	+	?
2	+	+	−	+	−	−	?
3	−	+	−	−	+	−	+
4	−	+	+	+	+	−	−

The reader need not be disturbed by the fact that this table is an artificial presentation. It is a condensed summary of a mass of data and shows that four distinct antibodies can be recognised, each displaying a consistent pattern of reactions with seven distinct antigens. The second antibody is anti-D (though it was not then so called) and the pattern of reactions indicates an association between these antibodies. The relationship of the first and fourth antibodies is particularly direct for their reactions are the opposite of each other.

From this last observation Sir Ronald Fisher deduced that the antigens being recognised by these two antibodies were mutually exclusive. In other words the genes determining these antigens were alleles (like D and d) so that one or other, but not both, could be inherited from a parent and occupy the appropriate site on the chromosome. He called these two alleles, and the antigens they determine, C and c, no doubt because A and B were already in use as blood group symbols.

Having explained the reactions of the first and fourth antibodies in this way, Fisher supposed that, as the reactions of the second and third antibodies were not opposite to each other, two further antibodies might be encountered having reactions antithetical to numbers 2 and 3. And so it proved. Fisher's predictions were soon confirmed and the two antibodies having the reactions expected of them, were apparently discovered. These six antibodies were recognising six antigens which Fisher called C and c, D and d and E and e. Each person might inherit one of each of these three pairs from one parent (it might be CDe for example) and another trio from the other parent. Thus the antigenic structure, or genotype, of a single individual might be expressed, thus, CDe/cDE as an example.

The seven sets of antibody reactions given in Table III were thus seven of the eight possible combinations of CcDdEe ; and Fisher again successfully predicted the discovery of the eighth combination which was found in a sample of cells a few years later. The completed set of reactions is given in Table IV in which the antigens and antibodies are given the names they now bear. The evidence on which Fisher's predictions were based is surrounded by a line.

It is necessary to pause at this point to examine the situation as it appeared in the late 1940's. It appeared that an individual might inherit from each parent a complex of three Rh genes, and that each of these genes would be one of a pair of alleles, C or c, D or d and E or e. No question has arisen about the Cc or Ee pairs ; nor is

TABLE IV

Antibodies	Genes and antigens							
	CDe	cDE	cde	cDe	cdE	Cde	CDE	CdE
Anti-C	+	−	−	−	−	+	+	+
Anti-D	+	+	−	+	−	−	+	−
Anti-E	−	+	−	−	+	−	+	+
Anti-c	−	+	+	+	+	−	−	−
(Anti-d)	(−)	(−)	(+)	(−)	(+)	(+)	(−)	(+)
Anti-e	+	−	+	+	−	+	−	−

there any doubt about D. But now, some ten years later, doubt has arisen about anti-d.

One cannot now be certain that the existence of d and anti-d has been unequivocally demonstrated. Despite much work and experiment no samples of anti-d have come to light in recent years. One may take the view that d does not exist. Or, knowing that c and e do exist, one may say that d is bound to turn up sooner or later as so many other predicted blood groups have done. And one may be so impressed by the symmetry displayed by blood group genes that hope for the discovery of d may still be sustained. But at present the existence of d is not proved. The reader may feel that he has been the victim of a deceit in that the whole argument has been built on the existence of d and the nature of its difference from D. But what is doubtful about D and d is perfectly certain about E and e or C and c, or, for that matter, any other blood group systems to be discussed. The presumption of d's existence is a matter of convenience in exposition and will be maintained, but it is necessary always to bear in mind that the existence of d is not proved.

A general element of doubt should also be voiced at this point. All that is said in this chapter about the Rh complex represents a working hypothesis widely accepted for some years. Some recent observations, not entirely consistent with this hypothesis, have cast some doubt over the matter. But this hesitation should not prevent the reader from enjoying this exposition until a substantially revised synthesis becomes generally accepted.

One may turn now to a consideration first of the consequences that flow from Fisher's synthesis and then of the additional alleles more recently discovered.

Fisher's synthesis at once simplifies and explains what might otherwise appear a complex series of reactions. It is based on the view that there are three closely-situated but independent sites on the chromosome (loci) which will receive one of each pair of alleles. The closeness of the loci, as well as their independence, can be illustrated by examining further evidence.

The loci are regarded as closely-situated because the three antigens are not inherited independently, but as a complex ; a Cde/Cde parent, for example, would be capable of handing on only Cde. This is another way of saying that genetical crossovers do not occur between these sites, and as crossing-over occurs commonly between genes that are not close together, it can be assumed that these sites are indeed close. Indeed no cross-over has ever been detected between these sites, no case having been encountered of a person having a combination not found in either of his parents. The evidence of Table V, however, suggests that cross-overs do occasionally occur between these loci.

Before examining Table V it is desirable to recall that the labels C, D and E arose arbitrarily, influenced by the order of discovery ; there was no reason to suppose that this represented the order of loci on the chromosome. In fact, as will be supported by evidence in the ensuing paragraphs, there is reason to believe the order to be DCE. Since the order is probably DCE and since D is the most important of the antigens it would be a small, but rational and desirable, step towards the improvement of notation if all genotypes were expressed in this order. This practice is already gaining ground and will be followed here.

TABLE V

DCe	40·8 per cent.
dce	38·9 ,, ,,
DcE	14·1 ,, ,,
Dce	2·6 ,, ,,
dcE	1·2 ,, ,,
dCe	1·0 ,, ,,
DCE	0·2 ,, ,,
dCE	exceedingly rare

Table V shows the approximate incidence of the eight Rh antigen complexes in Britain, and it will be observed that there are three orders of frequency; those that are relatively common, 12 per cent. or over, those of 3 per cent. or less and finally dCE of exceptional rarity. If cross-overs occur among the three common complexes where the dotted line is placed then the four combinations of the second order of frequency would arise.

```
D   d          D   d
.........
C   c   gives  c + C
e   e          e   e

D   D          D   D
C   c   gives  C + c
.........
e   E          E   e

D   d          D   d
c   c   gives  c + c
.........
E   e          e   E
```

Occasional cross-overs, therefore, occurring in the common complexes would furnish those that are less common and, as in each of the three cross-overs postulated, Dce (or cDe) results, one might suppose that it would occur about three times as commonly in the population as the other complexes of the second order of frequency. Reference to Table V shows this to be so. The rarity of dCE may be explained by its formation being possible only by a cross-over involving one of the less common complexes, and hence it could be expected that its incidence would be extremely low. It should be made clear that these calculations apply to the population as a whole, and no cross-over in any particular family has been detected.

For what this evidence is worth it does support the view that the three loci, though very close, are occasionally separable by cross-overs. A further piece of evidence suggests that the loci, though close, are independent. This was the discovery of a sample of blood in which no representative of the C or E loci could be detected. It suggested that a small piece of chromosome normally carrying the C and E loci had disappeared from this subject and only the D locus remained. This sample of blood was called — D —/— D — as an expression of its genotype, though perhaps it should now be D — —/D — — ; the fact that the patient was homozygous in this peculiar respect was due to the interrelationship of her parents who were half second cousins. A similar chromosome deletion has been reported from America in which the E locus was missing. These deletions support strongly the presumed order DCE ; and the evidence generally implies that the D site is not as close to C as C is to E.

Recently evidence has arisen to suggest that another locus exists for which the alleles have been called F and f. The order is almost certainly DCEF. There is yet another antigen whose place in the system is not yet clear—it may be part of a further pair of alleles, which have been called, temporarily, V and v ; V is common in negroes and rare in white persons. V and f have been identified, but the presumed v and F await discovery.

One may picture, therefore, a short segment of chromosome upon which there are four, perhaps five, gene loci linearly disposed and very close together ; the first of the loci will carry D or d and the other three in order will carry C or c, E or e and F or f respectively. The Rh blood group system might be described genetically as comprising four closely-linked and adjacent loci for which four pairs of alleles compete. This picture is a likely deduction rather than a proved fact ; and in due course V and v might be incorporated.

The sequence of these observations, and the adoption of a notation using small and capital letters may give rise to an erroneous impression that the normal number of alleles available for each gene locus is two. In fact there are more. There may be perhaps three or four variant forms of C, of which C and c may possibly represent the opposite extremes. These other alleles are distinguished by superscript symbols, *e.g.* C^u, C^v. These variants are of no great practical importance, but they are of sufficient interest in other respects to be worth a brief mention.

The alleles at the C locus that are at present known are called C, C^u, C^w, C^x, c^v and c. Of these C^w is the only variant, apart from C and c, that is not rare. It is called C^w rather than c^w because its properties are very similar to C. The existence of anti-C^w antibodies (*i.e.* those reacting with C^w but not with C or c) is well attested, and in one case at least this antibody has caused hæmolytic disease of the newborn. Since both anti-C and anti-C^w are known, it would be reasonable to suppose that C and C^w are distinct substances even though they are related. But antibodies reacting with *both* C and C^w are common and appear to arise from immunisation with C alone. These antibodies are, for convenience, called anti-C + C^w, but they do not appear to be mixtures of independent antibodies, for they cannot be separated by absorption (as, for example, a mixture of anti-C + anti-D can). This curious fact has been explained by supposing that the two antibody groupings are carried on the one molecule : but this view is capable of unjustifiable extension which might raise serious difficulties. It might be wiser at present to regard the difference between C and C^w as a slight chemical one so that most antibodies are capable of reacting effectively with both forms ; but that some antibodies are able to react only with C and others only with C^w. Those antibodies that react with both forms do so more effectively with C than with C^w.

The other alleles at this locus may be dealt with more briefly. C^x is very rare and may be recognised by a specific anti-C^x antibody and by some samples of anti-C. C^u may be regarded, for simplicity, as a rather weaker form of C ; it is recognised by some, but not all anti-C sera. The most interesting perhaps is c^v. It is agglutinated by some samples of anti-C and some of anti-c. It may therefore be thought of as having certain components of both C and c. This forms a marked contrast with D antigens ; C and c may not be so very dissimilar if some of their properties can be combined in c^v, but D and d are so dissimilar that the former is an antigen so powerful that it is responsible for hæmolytic disease of the newborn, whereas d is so weakly antigenic that its very existence has been questioned.

The variation that occurs at the D locus seems to be constant in kind but different in degree. The variation takes the form of a rather weaker reaction to anti-D. To be more precise, the variant cells, which are called D^u, react with some but not all anti-D sera and are discovered better by the antiglobulin reaction than by other techniques. D^u could, at present, be regarded as a weaker form of D, possibly due simply to there being fewer antigens on each red cell. Not all samples of D^u exhibit the same *degree* of weakness, some being less reactive than others ; the degree of weakness, however, seems to be precisely inheritable. D^u is rare but is important because without adequate tests the D^u could be missed and the subject classed as d. This error could lead to the administration of D^u blood to a d person with the result that the recipient might form anti-D. A very rare experience, which is less easy to explain is the formation of anti-D by some D^u persons.

The alleles at the E locus are all rare (apart from E and e) and do not display any points of principle different from those at the other loci. Three have been discovered, termed E^u, E^w and e^x.

It is not intended that anything should be said here about certain genetical aspects of these closely-linked loci such as the effect of position on the expression of the genes or the interference by some genes in the expression of others, but there is one point of this kind which may prove of considerable practical importance. There is some evidence that D is more antigenic when in the combination DcE than in DCe. There is more than one possible explanation for this, but its practical significance is that Rh positive fathers having an E are more likely to immunise their wives against D, and have more severely affected babies, than those with C.

The question of compatibility for blood transfusion needs further consideration in the light of these Rh complexes. The administration of D blood into a person lacking D is likely to give rise to antibody formation, whereas the transfusion of d blood into a person lacking this antigen is harmless. The transfusion of C or E blood into cc or ee persons is also undesirable though neither of these substances is as antigenic as D. Nor is administration of c or e blood into CC or EE persons entirely without risk and both anti-c and anti-e may be encountered, more particularly the former. It follows that the administration of rhesus negative blood (dce/dce) to rhesus positive persons is potentially dangerous and should not be done ill-advisedly. For most practical purposes D is the antigen that matters, but it is as well to bear in mind that the other members of the Rh complex (except d) may occasionally give rise to antibody formation.

CHAPTER VI

SOME MINOR GROUPS AND THEIR NOTATION

In any rapidly expanding branch of science there is always considerable difficulty and often confusion in trying to devise a system of nomenclature that can be extended to incorporate later discoveries without invalidating the names invented to explain the earlier observations; and in trying to use names or symbols that reflect the observed evidence with reasonable accuracy without carrying unjustified implications about properties that have not been tested or proved. Blood-group nomenclature and notation have proved particularly troublesome in this way. It will be seen that new knowledge has already outgrown the inflexible nomenclature that was originally adopted for the ABO and MN blood group systems; and in these only ingenious variation can be employed in the hope of diminishing confusion. The Rh system of nomenclature has been most ably devised and ingeniously extended so as to allow of a simple grasp of what could be a most complex assembly of antigens. Even so there are difficulties; the employment of capital and small letters falsely implying a genetical dominance and recessiveness is but one example, and there are others; what was first called CDE one would now like to call DCE, the justification of thinking of C^w as a variant of C, when it may be the other way round, or of using lower case for c^v when it may react with anti-C and having only one symbol, D^u, for several variants.

These may not be thought serious defects, and their appraisal is not intended as a commentary upon the difference of opinion between Dr. Wiener and other experts concerning whether the DCE notation should be used at all, or instead a system of capital R's printed in various ways and attended by a number of superscript and subscript signs. As to this dispute, it is of no consequence to anyone but those who aspire to those intellectual levels at which it is conducted, and they may judge for themselves; the rest may be content to adopt whichever system best stands the test of time.

But the discovery of each new blood group raises essentially the same problem afresh and an attempt has been made to devise a system flexible enough to allow the necessary expansion, and yet reasonably consistent between one blood group system and another. Such a scheme may now be set out in its application to one blood group system as an example. The blood group *Duffy* is chosen.

This group receives its name from the patient on whom investigations led to its discovery, and with his permission. It was not possible to use D or Du as shorthand symbols for this group because these or similar symbols were bespoken in the Rh system; hence Fy was adopted. The differentiation of alleles by small and capital letters was avoided and the symbols Fy^a and Fy^b used instead. This has the advantage of not implying any dominance or other inequality between them, and a further 24 alleles could be discovered without embarrassing the notation by running out of superscript letters. The genes, then, that can be inherited are Fy^a and Fy^b, which may be homozygous as in Fy^aFy^a or Fy^bFy^b, or heterozygous as in Fy^aFy^b. If an anti-Fy^a antibody alone is used to examine red cells the results are expressed thus, Fy(a +) or Fy(a —), for all that this test could disclose is the presence or absence of the antigen Fy^a. If it is present, Fy(a +), one cannot say whether the cells are homozygous or heterozygous; if it is absent, Fy(a —), one has not direct evidence that Fy^b is present until the cells are tested with anti-Fy^b. When both antibodies are used the results are expressed thus ; homozygous Fy^a cells would be Fy(a + b —), but heterozygotes, reacting with both sera, would be Fy(a + b +), and finally those cells reacting only with anti-Fy^b would be Fy(a — b +).

By way of summary the notations may be listed thus :

Group	Duffy
Known genes	Fy^a and Fy^b
Possible genotypes	Fy^aFy^a or Fy^aFy^b or Fy^bFy^b
Phenotypes determined by use of one antibody	Fy(*a* +) or Fy(a —)
Phenotypes determined using both antibodies	Fy(a + b —) or Fy(a + b +) or Fy(a — b +)

This table illustrates the uses of the terms phenotype and genotype. Phenotype is merely a convenient word for referring to such information as is available about the genetic structure with the means that are at the investigator's disposal. If he has only anti-Fy^a available and the cells do not react with this, he can justifiably express the result only as the phenotype Fy(a —) ; as far as is at present known the genotype of such a sample is likely to be Fy^bFy^b but without testing with anti-Fy^b or investigating other members of the family one could not be sure that there may not be an Fy^c hitherto undiscovered. Where family studies or other evidence can certainly determine the genetic structure, then the term genotype is used.

In addition genes and antigens may be distinguished in all groups by setting the symbols in italic when referring to genes and in roman when referring to antigens.

The Duffy Group (discovered in 1950)

The incidence of the Fy^a antigen is about 66 per cent. and that of Fy^b is about 34 per cent. It may be that Fy^a is more antigenic than Fy^b, because many samples of anti-Fy^a have been encountered but only a few of anti-Fy^b. Anti-Fy^a reacts poorly or not at all by direct agglutination or by the albumin or trypsin tests, but is effective if the antiglobulin test is used. A few transfusion reactions have been reported as due to this antibody. Most negroes have neither Fy^a nor Fy^b, but no antibody has yet been discovered that identifies a third allele at this locus.

Lutheran (discovered in 1946)

The short symbol for this group is Lu. Both anti-Lu^a and anti-Lu^b are rare and the group is not important medically.

Kell (discovered in 1946)

The antigen K was discovered in Britain, and k was discovered independently in America, being at first called Cellano. (The names in most of these groups are taken from the patient in whom the antigen or antibody was first found.) The antigen k is almost universal, having an incidence of 99·8 per cent., and Kell positive people are nearly all heterozygous (*i.e.* KK is a very rare combination). A number of samples of both anti-K and anti-k are known ; either may cause hæmolytic disease of the newborn but the former is far the more dangerous. K is, in fact, quite a powerful antigen and this group must be reckoned with in clinical practice. The newly discovered antibodies, anti-Kp^a and anti-Kp^b have disclosed two new antigens closely related to K and k.

KIDD (discovered in 1951)

The short symbols for the alleles of the Kidd group are Jk^a and Jk^b. Several samples of antibodies against both antigens have been found ; they react best by the anti-globulin reaction. The incidence is approximately 76 per cent Jk^a and 74 per cent. Jk^b.

New blood groups are being discovered astonishingly frequently. Some are so rare that no examples are found outside the families of the patients in whom they were first discovered. Others, after a period of independent existence, are shown to be related to one of the existing systems. Some recently discovered antigens whose progress may be worth watching are Wr^a, Di^a, Yt^a, Vel and Js^a.

CHAPTER VII

THE MNS SYSTEM

It is at this stage that the reader may appreciate the decision to present a summary of knowledge of human blood groups in the order that has been selected. The evidence that has been discussed so far about the serological behaviour of blood group antigens and antibodies has been consistent with the known properties of antigens and antibodies generally, and such variations as have been noted have been easy to comprehend and assess. Likewise the inheritance of blood-group antigens can be explained, on the evidence so far presented, as dependent on a number of allelic genes competing for certain chromosome loci, and that in the Rh group there are three or four known loci closely adjacent. It is again true to say that such few variations from this simple interpretation as are known do not seriously invalidate the basic concept. And for all these phenomena a reasonable attempt has been made to devise simple and, as far as possible, meaningful systems of notation and nomenclature. But in turning now to other blood groups, particularly those discovered before the Rhesus factor, some additional complications arise when recent discoveries have to be grafted on to an existing notation. Of this the MNS system provides an example.

The antigens M and N were first described in 1927, and were discovered in experiments on rabbit antisera prepared against human cells ; however, human examples of anti-M and anti-N are fully substantiated. M and N are alleles for a single locus so that, as usual, one can find homozygous persons, MM or NN, or heterozygous persons, MN.

Variants of M and N are known (called M_2 and N_2) and one, called M^c, is thought to be intermediate between M and N (in much the same way as c^v is thought to be intermediate between C and c). A recently discovered variant, called M^g, does not react with anti-M or anti-N.

Twenty years later the discovery of a certain antiserum led to the belief that there was another locus associated with the MN one, for which the two alleles were called S and s. This was confirmed in due course by the finding of anti-s to complete the picture sketched by anti-S. These two loci are close together so that cross-overs do not separate them ; the situation is comparable to that described for the Rh loci. It is far from convenient having the alleles of one locus labelled with two different capital letters (M and N) and those of the other locus distinguished by capital and small forms of the same letter (S and s), and the situation is worsened by the discovery of a third allele at this locus called S^u, which indicates lack of S or s. The approximate incidences of these groups in Britain are M 28 per cent, N 22 per cent., S 32 per cent. and s 89 per cent. The only one of these antigens that seems to be powerful enough to evoke antibody formation at all commonly is S. One may summarise the position by saying that there are two established loci in this system, the alleles of one of which being M, N and rarely M^g and of the other S, s and rarely S^u.

It is now necessary to find room for at least five new antigens in this system. Two of these, Hunter (Hu) and Henshaw (He) are more common in negroes than in white people and seem to be associated closely with N, and in the case of He, with S as well. The other two, Mi^a and Vw, are closely associated with each other as well as with MN and Ss. Of the latest, V^r, little is yet known.

This system is of very minor interest clinically, but it does illustrate how confused blood group notation may become. In 1927 it seemed as though the whole topic had been finished by the demonstration of the two alleles M and N ; and for twenty years this view, based on simple agglutination reactions, was not assailed by any newly-accruing evidence. But now, more than thirty years later, it has become a mass of arbitrary and, at first sight, unrelated symbols. Admittedly many of them are but temporary labels attached to the antigen until it can be assigned to its appropriate place in the system and a convenient and meaningful sign invoked. One may feel that a revised notation for all blood groups is becoming pressing. Such a revision will not inconvenience the clinician who encounters but a handful of these antigens in normal practice ; and the expert will be intellectually gratified and can always be furnished with a glossary. Perhaps the greatest impediment to a revision of the notation is fear of tackling the sacrosanct international nomenclature of the ABO system.

CHAPTER VIII

THE ABO SYSTEM

ALTHOUGH the ABO blood groups were the first by many years to be discovered and are the most important of all groups clinically, they display such unusual features, in comparison with other groups, that they are hardly a suitable introduction to the topic in general. As early as the year 1900 Karl Landsteiner showed that the human race could be divided into several groups by the agglutination reactions of red-blood cells, and these observations were rounded off by two of his pupils two years later. This is, perhaps, a convenient place to recall that Landsteiner, in addition to this great scientific contribution in 1900, discovered, with Levine, the M, N and P groups in 1927, and the Rh group, D, in 1940, this time with Wiener. He would no doubt be astonished were he able to witness the remarkable acceleration of blood-group discovery during the last decade.

The original observations at the beginning of the century showed that mankind could be divided into four groups which could be explained by supposing the existence of two different blood-group substances called A and B. In one group were placed those carrying one of these substances, A, on the red cells (Group A) and in the second, those carrying the other (Group B). The third group comprised those carrying both substances (Group AB) and the last group those carrying neither (Group O). A later discovery of a weaker variant of A, called A_2, increased the number of groups to six, viz., A_1, A_2, B, A_1B, A_2B and O.

The first peculiarity of the ABO system that merits

attention is the presence of natural antibodies. In all the blood-group systems so far discussed it has been assumed that no antibody will be present in a person's serum unless that person lacks the antigen concerned and has been subject to an antigenic stimulus that would provoke the formation of antibody. Indeed, this is general serological experience. But anti-A and anti-B arise spontaneously, in the absence of proved antigenic stimulus, during the first year of life. Of course the antibody does not appear in those carrying the same antigen, so that anti-A does not occur in persons who possess the A antigen, and is thus found in all persons belonging to Group B and Group O ; similarly anti-B occurs in persons of Group A and Group O. The antibody anti-A commonly has two components, which may be called anti-A and anti-A_1 ; the former agglutinates all A cells whether A_1 or A_2 ; but anti-A_1 agglutinates only A_1 cells and may, indeed, be found in persons of Group A_2 or A_2B. More will be said later of the features of anti-A.

In its simplest genetic form the ABO system may be regarded as resulting from the inheritance from each parent of one of four allelic genes at one locus, namely A_1, A_2, B and O. Persons belonging to Group A_1 may have one of three possible antigenic combinations, A_1A_1, A_1A_2, or A_1O ; and those belonging to group A_2 may be either A_2A_2 or A_2O. All that can be determined by the use of the available antisera (anti-A and anti-A_1) is the phenotype, *i.e.* A_1 or A_2. To determine the genotype, for example A_1A_2 or A_1O, it may be necessary to test several members of the family in the hope of deducing which genes are being handed on. An example of such deduction of genotypes from family studies is taken from Race and Sanger's book (pp. 19 and 20 of the third edition)—". . . in the first family . . . it is clear from the blood groups of the two elder children that each of the parents must possess an O gene. The father, therefore, is of the genotype BO and the mother A_1O. In the second family the father and the girl twin are of the phenotype A_1, and without the evidence provided by the genotypes of the mother and the boy twin their genotypes could not have been ascertained. The boy has received B from his mother and A_2 has come from his father, whose genotype must be A_1A_2. The girl of the phenotype A_1 has no B and must therefore have received A_2 from her mother ; the genotype of the girl twin is consequently A_1A_2."

First family

Father
Group B
[BO]

Mother
Group A
[AO]

son
Group O
[OO]

daughter
Group O
[OO]

son
Group AB

Second family

Father
Group A
[A_1A_2]

Mother
Group A_2B

twins

daughter
Group A
[A_1A_2]

son
Group A_2B

The genotypes of the other groups are more straightforward ; Group B persons must be either BB or BO, Group AB persons must be either A_1B or A_2B and Group O persons must all be OO. In Britain the frequencies of these groups is A 44·7 per cent. (A_1 34·8 per cent. and A_2 9·9 per cent.), B 8·6 per cent., AB 3·2 per cent. (A_1B 2·6 per cent. and A_2B 0·6 per cent.) and O 43·5 per cent.

A second peculiarity of the ABO system is that the antigenic substances A and B are found not only in the red cells but in the tissue cells and plasma as well ; moreover they are also secreted in the bodily secretions, such as saliva. But the formation of these blood-group substances on the cells and in the secretions is governed by a number of independently acting genes. One of these genes, called X, is necessary for the development of the B antigen both on the cells and in the secretions (it may also influence the A antigen, but of this we have no evidence). The lack of the X gene (*i.e.* inheritence of xx) thus causes failure of development of the B antigen in persons known to have received a B gene.

The second gene, Y, influences the development of the A antigen (but does not concern B) on the cells, but it does not modify the secretion of the A antigen. Therefore persons inheriting an A gene but lacking the Y gene are able to secrete it in their saliva, but do not seem able to put the A antigen on to their cells. The third gene is the secretor gene Se. About 76 per cent. of Europeans are either SeSe or Sese and can secrete the A and B substances in the saliva and bodily secretions, but those lacking Se (*i.e.* sese) can put the A and B antigens on their cells, without being able to secrete them.

By way of summary, therefore, there are, in addition to the genes responsible for the inheritance of the A and B substances, genes controlling the development of these substances on the cell and in the secretions. Without X (either in the homozygous or heterozygous state) a person cannot develop the B antigen on his cells or in his secretions, despite his having received the B gene. Without Y, the A antigen will not develop on the cells but may appear in the secretions, depending upon the presence of the Se gene which is necessary if these blood-group substances are to appear in the secretions.

It is as well at this stage to consider the gene O, a topic so obscure that it is almost impossible to say anything sensible about it. Persons of genetype OO must presumably inherit a gene of some kind even though all that can be said about it is that it is not A or B. The inheritance of the O gene does not lead to the development of an antigen that can provoke the formation of a specific antibody (*i.e.* one that agglutinates AO cells as well as OO cells). Yet a number of antisera are known that do agglutinate Group O cells but not those of Groups A_1 or B ; they usually also agglutinate cells of Group A_2. The source of most of these sera is not a human one and yet a few samples of human sera have been described that have these properties. One positive observation about these antisera has led to their being divided into two kinds ; some of them are not neutralised by the addition of saliva from a secretor person of whatever group, and these are called anti-O sera. The others are neutralised by saliva from secretors irrespective of their group and these are called anti-H.

One may picture the situation thus. Secretors have the H substance on their red cells whichever group they belong to, but it is, to some extent, superseded by the A and B substances when these are present. Hence anti-H sera do not agglutinate Group A or Group B cells, but are capable of agglutinating Group A_2 or Group O cells. Nevertheless there is sufficient H substance in the secretions of persons of all groups (if they are secretors) to neutralise anti-H. Non-secretors (sese) do not secrete H, though they have it on their cells. Probably the only people who do not have H on their cells are those lacking the gene X, and the first of such persons to be described (the " Bombay " type) had anti-H in the serum.

It is thus customary to refer to three genes, A, B and O, though the existence of the third gene as an entity that is something more than mere absence of A and B has not been proven. It is customary also to refer to three antigens A, B and H, the last probably being present in all cells though most manifest in those of Group O and only a little less so in those of Group A_2. Group O and Group A_2 cells may be agglutinated by certain antisera some of which are called anti-H (for they are neutralised by saliva from secretors) and the others, not so neutralised, are called anti-O. This account carefully evades any explicit statement about the relationship between the gene O and the antigen H.

From what has been said about H and O it may be realised that the relationship of A_1 to A_2 cannot easily be defined ; genetically they are alleles but serologically their relationship is obscure and it cannot unequivocably be classed as qualitative or quantitative. There are also a number of weaker forms of A of which A_3 is the best established. The B antigen also has certain weaker variants of no clinical importance, but a recent observation concerning this antigen is of interest. It has been shown that in some elderly sick patients who are not of Group B, a B-like antigen may be acquired temporarily on their cells. These cells in this state react with anti-B sera, but not with the patient's own anti-B antibodies. This matter awaits further enquiry. The A and B antigens also appear weaker at birth and during the first few weeks of life.

The Antibodies of the ABO System

It has already been mentioned that a peculiarity of the ABO system is the natural presence of anti-A and of anti-B in persons not possessing the corresponding antigen. It was no doubt the presence of these antibodies that led to the ABO blood groups' being the first to be discovered. It is also because of the existence of these antibodies that the ABO groups are more important in blood transfusion than are other blood groups. A single bottle of blood incompatible for A or B is likely to cause immediate trouble because the recipient has antibodies already present ; in other groups the antibodies have to be manufactured and difficulties may develop more slowly.

Anti-A and anti-B are weak or absent at birth, but make their appearance after a few months ; they reach their maximum strength by ten years of age. It is difficult to account for the natural occurrence of anti-A or anti-B in the sera of persons not possessing the corresponding antigen. Discussion has treated more fully the reason why anti-A or anti-B is absent from persons who do possess the corresponding antigen. It seems that if the fœtal tissues encounter *in utero* any potentially antigenic substance, that substance comes to be regarded as a natural component of the fœtus and hence not " foreign " and not antigenic. It has been suggested that the antibody-forming apparatus in fœtal life is learning to recognise, perhaps by codes, the fœtal tissues themselves, including the blood-group substances, so that antibodies are not produced by an organism against its own tissues. Indeed an animal may be rendered unable to produce antibodies in adult life against substances introduced to it in fœtal life, a state called " immunological tolerance." Immunological tolerance, therefore, develops to the A or B antigen inherited by the fœtus, and the natural antibodies appear only in the absence of the corresponding antigen. But why they appear at all has never been explained.

These natural antibodies (as they are called, but they may not be natural and are certainly unusual as antibodies) do not readily pass from mother to fœtus *in utero*, and do not give rise to hæmolytic disease of the newborn. There are, however, circumstances in which the properties of anti-A or anti-B may alter, and these changes result from immunisation of the patient by the A or B substances (*i.e.* by injection or transfusion of blood or blood products containing an antigen against which the patient already possesses a naturally-occurring antibody). It also appears that certain other vaccines (*e.g.* anti-tetanus inoculation) may bring about this change of character of anti-A or anti-B. The antibodies displaying these new properties are referred to as " immune " anti-A or anti-B and differ from their naturally-occurring counterparts in three important ways (and several minor ways). First, their *in vitro* activity is greater at body-heat than at room temperature ; (the reverse is true of the naturally-occurring antibodies which in this respect are unusual serologically). Secondly, they are capable of hæmolysing the appropriate cells *in vitro*, whereas the natural antibodies can do no more than agglutinate. Finally, the immune forms of anti-A and anti-B may reach the fœtus *in utero* and destroy fœtal cells ; they may thus be a cause of hæmolytic disease of the newborn.

Although it has been customary to refer to these antibodies as " immune " and " naturally-occurring " it has been shown that there is a difference of specificity. The immune form of anti-A which hæmolyses human A cells will also react with pig red cells of Group A, but the natural antibody does not. Moreover, pig group A cells can absorb the immune anti-A from an antiserum without altering the titre of the natural form. Hence it appears that a part of the human A antigen is also found in pig cells of Group A, and it is against this part that the immune anti-A is directed ; the other part of the human A antigen, which is not found in pig cells, is recognised by the natural form of anti-A.

The forms of antibody can thus be summarised : first, anti-A_1, a naturally-occurring room-temperature agglutinating antibody, specific for human A_1 cells. Second, anti-A, also a naturally-occurring room-temperature agglutinating antibody reacting with human A_1 and A_2 cells. Third, anti-A^p an immune, body-temperature hæmolysing antibody reacting with human and pig Group A cells. Less is known about anti-B.

There is reason to suppose that when anti-A and anti-B occur together in the same person (*i.e.* in Group O) their properties differ slightly from those when they are separate (as in Group A or Group B persons), or when artificially mixed from persons of the latter groups. In Group O sera there is some cross-absorption, *i.e.* some anti-B seems to be absorbed by A cells and *vice versa*, almost as if there were some antigenic component common to both groups and recognised by the sera of Group O persons, or some Group O persons, alone. It is also of interest, and may be relevant, that the immune forms of anti-A or anti-B giving rise to hæmolytic disease of the newborn seem to arise far more commonly in mothers of Group O than in those of Group A or B. Neither of these observations has yet been satisfactorily explained.

Hæmolytic Disease of the Newborn

Hæmolytic disease due to A or B differs in certain respects from the condition, already described, that results from Rh immunisation. Clinically there are no very great differences, though the disease due to anti-A or anti-B is usually milder (but it can be severe) and in its mild form may be quite common. Though the mechanism by which this disease comes about in ABO immunisation is not understood it clearly differs from that due to Rh immunisation. The naturally-occurring anti-A and anti-B do not seem to play much part, if any, in this disorder, and it is the formation of immune anti-A or B that causes trouble. The formation of these immune antibodies occurs very many times more frequently in Group O mothers than in those of Groups A or B. And there is no evidence that the immunising agent is an invasion of fœtal red cells following retro-placental hæmorrhage ; it is more likely to be the soluble blood group substance of the fœtus. Nor is parturition essential to the establishment of maternal immunisation and so first-born infants may be affected. Both secretor and non-secretor infants are liable. The antiglobulin test (or Coombs test) is a certain means of diagnosis of hæmolytic disease of all forms *except* that due to anti-A or anti-B. In all major respects other than those mentioned the disease is comparable, whether provoked by anti-D or anti-A or anti-B.

Incompatible Transfusion

The existence of the natural forms of anti-A and anti-B imposes a very strict practice upon blood transfusion if incompatibility and its consequences are to be avoided. It is most important to ensure that no red cells enter the circulation of a patient who carries an antibody against these cells. The most important antibodies to be ascertained and guarded against are anti-A and anti-B. If blood of Group A is infused into a person who carries anti-A the incoming cells will be rapidly destroyed by the patient's antibody. It is the destruction of transfused cells that constitutes the danger to the patient, for the disposal of such a large number of cells so rapidly cannot be accomplished without damage to the kidney which can, in severe cases, lead to death from the consequences of anuria.

It is necessary, therefore, always to administer blood of the same group as the patient's whenever this can be achieved. Normally this is accomplished in two stages. Firstly the ABO group of the patient is determined so that blood of the same group can be made available. Secondly, a " cross-match " is performed before the transfusion.

For this purpose some of the patient's serum is obtained and exposed to some cells from the particular sample of blood to be administered. This is to ensure that no antibodies are present in the patient's serum that would react with, and hence destroy, the transfused blood. This procedure is designed to cover all blood-group antibodies, not merely anti-A or anti-B, and it may be necessary, if the patient is thought to have antibody in the incomplete form, to perform the cross-match by some technique designed to reveal this form of antibody such as the albumin test or the antiglobulin test. In no circumstances should these two steps be omitted, and they should always be performed by a trained person in a properly-equipped laboratory ; bedside cross-matches can no longer be considered safe.

These steps provide against incompatible transfusion concerning anti-A, anti-B or other preformed antibodies in the patient, but they are not enough. It is necessary to ensure that the patient is not likely to become immunised by the proposed transfusion against blood-group antigens other than A or B. Of these the only one that is taken into account in routine transfusion is the Rh antigen D which is the most powerful, and hence the most troublesome, of the other blood-group antigens. For these reasons, and particularly because of the risk of subsequent hæmolytic disease in the children of female patients, it is essential to determine the Rh group (D or d) of the patient so that Rh compatible blood is administered. Neither of the first procedures given above ensures this.

To summarise, therefore : every patient requiring transfusion should have his cells examined for the antigens A, B and D. Blood of corresponding group should then be selected and a cross-match performed before it is administered. This represents the minimum safeguard which must be made available to every patient. Some patients require further careful and detailed preparation, for example those likely to receive repeated transfusions or otherwise suspected of an unusual predisposition to manufacture antibodies.

It is important that the idea does not gain ground that much of this preparation can be circumvented by administering blood of Group O dd indiscriminately. There are many reasons for this, of which a practical one is the difficulty the blood transfusion service would encounter in trying to meet a large demand for this far from common type of blood. But there is another reason which is worth comment. Incompatible transfusion has been described as the infusion of red cells containing an antigen against which the patient carries an antibody. It may be asked whether the infusion of antibodies into a patient carrying the corresponding antigen would also be dangerous ; these circumstances would arise if Group O blood (containing anti-A and anti-B) were given to someone of Group A, B or AB. Normally no ill-effects follow such a procedure, partly because the antibody is so diluted in the larger volume of the recipient's circulation that very few of the patient's red cells would be destroyed, but also because the incoming antibody would be neutralised by the soluble blood-group substances in the plasma. There are, however, rare occasions when Group O blood contains anti-A or anti-B in such high titre that its effect might be damaging to the patient's cells, particularly if the antibody is of the immune type. These rare samples are unsatisfactory for transfusion and have been called " dangerous universal donor " blood, a term that is now not very useful since the term " universal donor " has rightly been discarded. The initials " dud " might be retained, however.

It might be argued that in emergency when there may be no time or facilities for proper blood grouping of the patient, the administration of Group O dd blood might be justified. This argument is not strong. In the first place facilities for accurate blood grouping should always be available, day or night, wherever blood for transfusion is itself available. And as for time, there can be very few emergencies in which there is insufficient time, say half an hour, for the determination of blood group and cross-match; and most of these could be met by an initial infusion of some cell-free fluid such as plasma or dextran, while the blood-group work was being undertaken. The administration of blood of correct ABO and Rh group should be invariable in all cases requiring transfusion.

CHAPTER IX

P AND LEWIS

THE two remaining blood-group systems have been left till last because an appreciation of their properties depends on a knowledge of the ABO groups. The first of them, the P group, can be disposed of briefly. P was discovered in 1927, and, after the discovery in 1951 of the Jay system (short symbol Tj^a), it proved that they were related. It seems that the system is analagous to the ABO system and, by discarding the Tj notation, the P notation may be modelled on the ABO group as follows.

Those who have no P antigen, who may be referred to as pp, are analagous to Group O and have the naturally-occurring antibodies anti-P and anti-P_1 in their serum (just as Group O persons have anti-A and anti-A_1 in the serum). Such persons are extremely rare, indeed at present only fifteen are known in the world. Those who carry the P antigen may have it in one of two forms, P_1 or P_2, just as Group A persons have A_1 or A_2. Those belong to the subgroup P_1 (nearly 80 per cent. of persons in Europe) have no naturally-occurring anti-P in the serum, but those who are P_2 may have anti-P_1 (just as some A_2 persons have anti-A_1). Another antigen has recently been discovered in this system, called P^k.

The other blood-group system, called Lewis, displays a number of interesting features that are not found in other blood groups. It seems that two antigens can be recognised, called Le^a and Le^b, but about 6 per cent. of persons carry neither of these antigens. The incidence in adults of Le^a is about 22 per cent. and of Le^b is 72 per cent.; the incidence of Le^a is higher in children because children's cells heterozygous for Le^a are agglutinated but those from adults are not ; this unusual situation has not yet been explained.

The most notable feature about the Lewis group is a property that has not been found in any other human blood group, but is known in the J group in cattle and the R group in sheep. This is that the red cells are not furnished with the antigen directly but they absorb it from the plasma. This can also be accomplished *in vitro* ; cells lacking Le^a will become Le^a positive after exposure to plasma containing Le^a ; and the same can be shown for Le^b. Newborn infants lack the Lewis antigens at birth, but a few weeks later the antigens appear in the plasma and are absorbed on the cells. The genes that govern the development of these Lewis antigens, therefore, do not equip the red cells with the antigen but provide for its appearance in the plasma and in the bodily secretions such as saliva. The red cells then absorb the antigen on to their surface from the plasma in which, nevertheless, a good deal remains.

This genetical control of the secretion of blood-group substances into the plasma and saliva recalls the secretion of the A, B and H substances and there is a connection, though the genes governing Lewis secretion are not the same as those governing ABH secretion. A theory that meets most of the observed facts depends upon the premise that there is not usually enough soluble blood-group substance to provide an adequate amount of both ABH and Le^a antigen in the same person. Therefore a person carrying both the ABH secretor gene (Se) and the Le^a secretor gene (called L) cannot produce both substances and the ABH enjoys the preference. In other words, secretors of ABH are all Le^b. (If there were any surplus Le^a substance available in such persons it seems to go into the saliva and not the plasma, and hence not the red cells.)

Non-secretors of ABH (sese), on the other hand, leave plenty of soluble blood-group substance to be made into Le^a in persons possessing the Lewis secretor gene L, and all such persons are Le^a. Those who do not carry the Lewis secretor gene L are the 6 per cent. who are neither Le^a or Le^b. Possibly Table VI may help in appreciating these points, though it should be understood that much of this view is still speculative.

TABLE VI

Secretor genes for		Substances in	
ABH	Le^a	Saliva	Red cells (Lewis only)
+	+	ABH, (Le^a) Le^b	Le^b
—	+	Le^a	Le^a
+	—	ABH	none
—	—	none	none

This theory seems to leave Le^b in a rather anomalous position at present and it has even been suggested that there may be no Le^b gene. Anti-Le^b sera, too, display some curious features. Some of them agglutinate Le^b cells of Group A_2 or O but not those of Group A_1. This could be explained by suggesting that the A antigen may have used so much of the material available for the manufacture of soluble substance that there is a shortage not only of Le^a but also of Le^b in the plasma for red cells to absorb ; the shortage would not diminish the amount of Le^b in the saliva, and anti-Le^b sera of this type are all neutralised by the saliva of ABH secretors. But the other form of anti-Le^b, though more normal serologically, does not fit into this pattern. This latter agglutinates all Le^b-containing cells irrespective of ABO group.

CHAPTER X

BLOOD GROUPS AND DISEASE

The relationship of blood groups to hæmolytic disease of the newborn and to incompatible blood transfusion has already been discussed. These are the two principal ways in which blood groups can be a direct cause of disease : and of disease which is in large measure preventable. There are other ways, however, in which blood groups appear to be related to certain diseases though the mechanisms of the relationship are obscure. At present the means of enquiry into these matters is statistical.

Naturally the known relationship of blood groups to hæmolytic disease of the newborn has led to an examination of the possible role of blood groups in other forms of failure to bring pregnancy to full term, abortions and miscarriages, toxæmia of pregnancy and similar conditions, but without convincing association being demonstrated.

Another group of diseases that has been studied in this respect is disorder of the upper part of the intestinal tract, peptic ulcer, gastric cancer and pernicious anæmia. It must be remembered that the soluble blood group substances are secreted from the gastric mucosa (which is affected in these disorders) as well as from the salivary glands which have also been studied with this in mind. In all these disorders an association with blood groups has been revealed.

Disease of the stomach and duodenum occupies the central place. Peptic ulceration of all kinds is significantly commoner in persons of Group O, both in many parts of Europe and in widely-scattered parts of the world. The association is even more pronounced with duodenal ulcer than with gastric ulcer. It is also clear that ulceration is much commoner in non-secretors of the ABO blood group substances ; it is probably more common in those whose gastric HCl secretion is promoted by histamine. There are no means at present of interpreting these results, but one cannot help wondering if the secretion into the stomach of the A or B substance may not afford some protection against peptic ulceration—particularly of the duodenum. This view is no more than guess-work.

Two other diseases of the stomach show a different association ; they are cancer of the stomach and pernicious anæmia (true pernicious anæmia arising primarily from atrophy of the gastric mucosa). Both of these conditions are commoner in persons of Group A though the secretor status of sufferers from these disorders has not yet been determined. It may be that the actual site of the gastric lesion (both with ulceration and cancer) is more particularly related to blood group influences and this, to be speculative again, may be concerned with the distribution of secretory activity in different parts of the stomach. It has been suggested that Group A predominates in both cancers and ulcers when the lesion is in the antrum and that Group O predominates when the lesion is in the body ; if this were so the association of cancer with Group A and ulcers with Group O may merely reflect the higher incidence of cancers in the antrum and ulcers in the body. Another form of tumour in a tissue of the upper alimentary tract that secretes blood group substance has also been shown to be commoner in Group A, namely salivary gland tumours.

One further condition that has been found to be commoner in persons of Group A also concerns a gland in the upper alimentary tract, but in the endocrine portion of it, so the question of secretion of the blood-group substances does not seem to be relevant. This condition is diabetes mellitus, a genetical predisposition to which has long been suspected.

There are other disorders in which an association with blood groups is suspected and there is little doubt that still more will be found and confirmed. There are, too, a number of diseases which can be shown not to be related to blood groups ; this is true of cancers of colon, rectum, lung and breast, of toxæmia of pregnancy and hypertension. All these studies relate to the ABO system, and despite several investigations no disorder, other than hæmolytic disease, has been shown to be related to Rh groups.

There are, finally, two other forms of disorder which display certain features relating to blood-group matters and which may provide useful evidence in future investigations. One of these is acquired hæmolytic anæmia in some forms of which an antibody active against the patient's own cells has been demonstrated. In some of these cases the antibody has been shown to be directed against a known antigen, such as the e antigen of the Rh system. The other form of disorder is systemic lupus erythematosus, and like conditions in which, it has been suggested, the patient may be more readily able to manufacture blood-group antibodies than is normal.

There is also evidence that very rarely the reactivity of the A or B antigens may be modified by serious disease. The temporary acquisition of a weak B-like antigen in sick or aged persons not of this group has already been mentioned. In other cases of severe bone marrow disease (myeloid leukæmia and hypoplastic anæmia) the A antigen on the cells has been found to be diminished in reactivity with specific antisera.

CHAPTER XI

BLOOD GROUPS AND GENETICS

THE study of human inheritance is rendered difficult by two sets of circumstances. Firstly, the number of generations available for study can only be few and the size of families often small ; there is no means of evading this problem at present. Second, many heritable characteristics are determined by complexes of genes which may be difficult to analyse. In the study of blood groups, however, the geneticist has a tool that is remarkably free from the latter disadvantage.

The usefulness of blood groups in genetical investigation is due to several features. It seems that in nearly every case the influence of a single gene determines one discernible effect, namely the development of a blood-group antigen. Moreover, there appears to be a minimal amount of extraneous interference with the power of the gene to bring about its effect, either from other genes situated nearby on the same chromosome, or from environmental factors generally. The study of blood-group antigens is therefore a very direct form of study of gene action. A large number of blood groups are now known, and so, since there are but 23 pairs of chromosomes in man, it may soon be possible to learn something about the positioning of these genes on the chromosomes and hence use them as markers to map out the site of other heritable characters.

Already, blood-group studies have furnished much information about mechanisms of inheritance. The concept of closely-linked adjacent loci found in the Rh and MNS systems is of fundamental interest and allows further consideration of cross-overs and their frequency. And the deletion of part of the chromosome, resulting in the D — — character, throws further light on genetical mechanisms. Again, the recent accumulation of knowledge about the secretor genes has enlightened our views about gene action and the organisation of basic material available to receive the imprint of the gene.

There are other genetical phenomena which may be illuminated by further investigation of blood groups. The forms of interference in the expression of genes by the effect of neighbouring genes, or other mechanisms of modification of gene expression, will no doubt find examples in blood groups. The effect, too, of blood groups and disease on the community will merit much study. If common diseases tend to diminish the survival of persons of certain groups a gradual change in blood-group frequencies would be expected if there were no compensating mechanism. The comprehension of such compensation would be a material contribution to the study of genetics.

A start has been made on the search for linkage between blood-group genes and other heritable characters. It seems quite clear that none of the existing blood groups is linked (*i.e.* carried nearby on the same chromosome) with any other blood group or with the sex character. These blood-group genes, therefore, represent the first reference points on what one day may become a map of gene positions on each chromosome. So far only three linkages with blood-group characters have been detected ; they are : (*a*) an association between the Lutheran gene and secretor genes ; (*b*) one between the Rh genes and that determining the production of oval red cells ; and (*c*) between the ABO genes and a rare condition, the nail-patella syndrome. Many more such linkages are to be expected. There are, too, other heritable characters that might assist in mapping the chromosomes, such as the ability to taste phenylthio-carbamide, the form of hæmoglobin and haptoglobin and the presence of certain substances in the serum or in the urine.

Knowledge of blood-group inheritance now permits the use of blood groups in problems of identity or disputed parentage. So long as the tests are adequately performed by an experienced worker there is no doubt whatever that incontrovertible evidence can be made available. If a child possesses a blood group not present in its reputed parents, then one of them has not engendered the child. It is this negative process of excluding parentage that is the most valuable contribution that blood groups can make ; and each additional blood-group system that is employed increases the chances that evidence could be made available that would exonerate a man wrongfully accused of paternity, as the following table, modified from Race and Sanger, shows :

TABLE VII

System	percentage exclusion summated
ABO alone	17·6
+ MNSs	37·3
+ Rh	53·1
+ Kell	54·9
+ Lutheran	56·4
+ Duffy	58·5
+ Kidd	59·7

Thus nearly 60 per cent. of falsely accused men could be exonerated if the alleged parents and the child were blood-grouped by all these systems ; and possibly this figure could be raised by employing other characters such as secretion. These investigations rarely achieve positive evidence of parentage, but even this might on occasions be possible if a rare combination of blood groups was concerned. There are less litigious uses of blood groups, however, in identifying babies that might have become attached to the wrong mothers in a maternity unit, or in distinguishing identical (monozygotic) twins, whose blood groups would be identical, from dizygotic twins whose blood groups would be likely to differ.

A discovery of the greatest interest that has been made about twins in recent times concerns the so-called chimeras. It has been known for some time that most dizygotic cattle twins have not completely separate placentas, with the consequence that the twins share some embryonic tissues between them in varying proportions. Hence some tissues destined for one twin become implanted in the other and develop successfully, and vice versa. Each twin, therefore, carries two sets of blood-group antigens, and, in the case of heifers, the endocrine mix-up results in sterility, the animal being termed a freemartin. Freemartins have not been observed in the human species, but cases of dizygotic twins with double blood-group systems have been reported, and called chimeras.

The following list gives the blood groups of the twins concerned in the first chimera to be discovered. The list on the left comprises the blood-group inheritance of the patient examined ; that on the right of the twin who had died twenty-five years before the investigation ; hence the groups are determined from the surviving twin, some 40 per cent. of her cells being, in effect, derived from primitive hæmopoietic tissue destined for her brother but implanted in her during embryonic life. The differences are confined to the ABO, Kell and Kidd systems.

O	A_1
MN.Ss	MN.Ss
P_1	P_1
CDeF/CDeF	CDeF/CDeF
Lu(a −)	Lu(a −)
kk	Kk
Le(a − b +)	Le(a − b +)
Fy(a +)	Fy(a +)
Jk(a + b +)	Jk(a − b +)

One of the features of interest in chimeras is the demonstration of "immunological tolerance." If foreign tissue becomes implanted in the embryo it becomes absorbed into the embryo as part of itself so that, in later life, when the foreign substance is again encountered, it is no longer recognised as foreign and antibodies are not made against it. The group O person above did not have any anti-A in the serum because of the implantation of A tissue in embryonic life. One would expect, therefore, that homografts between chimera twins would take despite the genetical dissimilarity, and this has been tried—successfully, so far—on one of the two pairs of chimera twins reported after the one described above.

CHAPTER XII

BLOOD GROUPS AND ANTHROPOLOGY

THE observations in the last chapter concerning human blood-group genetics, together with those of the preceding chapter concerning the relationship of blood groups to disease, lead to a consideration of whether blood groups can contribute to the study of mankind. These genetic markers may be expected to remain fairly constant in isolated breeding groups, except for the influence of disease on survival and fertility and hence on the composition of the population. If the various races or population masses of the world differ in their blood-group distribution it might be that blood-group studies in different parts of the world would throw some light on the history of man.

It is certainly true that blood-group distribution varies very widely from one part of the world to another, and a start has been made to estimate blood-group frequencies the world over. No time should be lost in making the survey as widespread and as detailed as possible, for modern conditions tend to the dispersal of what may well have been static or at least exclusive breeding groups over many hundreds of years.

In Europe, for example, some very rough distinctions emerge from the mass of data already accumulated. An arbitrary division following approximately the Iron Curtain leaves a very high incidence of B (10 per cent. or more) to the east but a high incidence of A to the west. A is particularly high in the Alpine region which may represent the cradle of one of the prehistoric groups of European settlers which later peopled the continent and is represented in Britain by Nordic immigrants. The successive waves of invaders falling on the rich and accessible south and east of these islands is today reflected by a higher incidence of Group A in these regions (cf. Sussex, 29 per cent., parts of Scotland 20–21 per cent.). And the mountainous refuges of the retreating Celts and Britons is reflected in a higher incidence of Group O detectable throughout a broad peripheral arc stretching from North Wales, and Ireland, through Scotland and its Western Islands to Iceland (cf. North Wales 68–72 per cent., Kent 64 per cent.).

The blood-group analysis of even smaller areas yields results of interest. In Wales, for example, in addition to the Celtic legacy of high O there may be detected a high B component in some areas where collateral evidence would support the view that this represents a contribution from another ancient race. An unexpected area of high A on the Pembroke peninsular coincides with a known Viking settlement.

Northern Europe poses many historical problems. The Celtic distribution of blood groups in Iceland questions the fate of the later Scandinavian invasions of this island. The Lapps also are evidently racially distinct, for their Eskimo neighbours do not share their high incidence of Group A_2, nor their Russian neighbours their low M.

Another distinctive race of interest is that of the Basques in the Pyrenees. This isolated community does not speak an Indo-European language and may, therefore, represent a stock established in Europe before the arrival of the earliest known Aryan hordes from the east. Their blood-group pattern supports this view, for their high O and low B differs from other invading groups, and in particular the incidence of d is higher among the Basques than anywhere else in the world. The gene d, being less common than D, is slowly being eliminated from all populations by the effect of hæmolytic disease of the newborn which threatens only heterozygotes (Dd) ; though there may be some compensatory genetic trend.

The high O and low B of the Basques contrasts with the great tongues of low incidence of O and high B radiating from the Caspian Sea which may represent the routes of invasion by the Asiatic peoples into Europe during the last two thousand years. The limit of their effective penetration is marked by the sharp decline of the incidence of B from 10 per cent. to the west of a line running south from the Gulf of Bothnia and the Baltic Sea along part of the river Elbe to the head of the Adriatic Sea. The high B is also characteristic of the Balkan peoples (except Greeks) and is found in the eastern Mediterranean and Egypt.

The Mediterranean basin, representing as it does the melting pot of many civilisations over many hundreds of years, shows a complex picture as might be expected. There is undoubtedly a contribution from the north European peoples with high A and fairly high B ; and also from the Basque progenitors with high O and d and low B. There is also a most distinctive component represented at this time by Sardinian stock who have a low incidence of A, B and d, together with a high M. Finally, there is a negro component bringing the specific Rh combination Dce and possibly the gene D^u.

It is to the land bridges into this basin from the south and east that one must look for migratory evidence ; unfortunately, in Turkey and the Levant the data are as yet incomplete. In Egypt a picture broadly intermediate between the Mediterranean example of Sardinia and the African findings can be detected. Indeed if the Rh groups alone are compared a surprisingly constant fall of D and D^u together with a rise in C can be observed in passing from East Africa via Egypt to Sardinia. This picture implies a passage of negro peoples along the Nile valley towards the Mediterranean, but the analysis of other blood groups shows this to be only a part of the story. In Cyprus the distinctive origin of the Greek-speaking and Turkish-speaking elements is not substantiated by blood groups.

The Sahara desert is shown to have been an effective barrier between the peoples of the Mediterranean littoral and the inhabitants of the rest of the African continent. Though the various African tribes display smaller differences between themselves, the peoples of this continent are as a whole characterised by a high incidence of Dce, P and Jk^a and a low one of S and Fy^a. In addition, certain antigens are found almost exclusively in African peoples ; S^u, He and Hu of the MNS system, and a recently discovered antigen Js^a.

The detailed observations of blood-group incidence elsewhere in the world show much complexity. In Asia the B gene shows a very high incidence, and in the south a high M is also found. Both of these genes show a fall as one passes towards the east, the B gradually (so that it is absent from Australian aborigines and very low in the Maori), the M suddenly, along Wallace's line, to be replaced to the eastward by a high incidence of N. In the extreme east, in China, A_2, d and P have disappeared but Fy^a is high. A recently discovered antigen, Diego (Di^a) seems to be characteristic of Mongoloid races.

Several distinctive populations have been studied such as the Australian aborigines (who have no B and very little S), the Ainu who differ markedly from their Japanese neighbours, and the Polynesians whose relationship with American aboriginal peoples betrays a common origin which is not inconsistent with Heyerdahl's theories ; though the blood-group evidence does not identify the first location of these peoples. The blood groups of Indians of the American continent very strongly suggest an Asiatic origin.

CHAPTER XIII

SOME GROWING POINTS

THE specialised techniques needed to investigate the chemical composition of blood-group antigens marks out this study as one distinct from the general run of blood group research. For the purposes of chemical analysis the blood-group substances concerned may be obtained from erythrocytes, from hog gastric mucosa or from certain bodily secretions, notably human ovarian cyst fluid. Hitherto the antigens most closely studied have been A, B, H and Le^a. They appear to contain carbohydrate and polypeptide as part of the same molecule. The carbohydrate moiety comprises four sugars, D-galactose, L-fucose, D-glucosamine and D-galactosamine. In the polypeptide moiety at least eleven amino acids have been identified. The specificity of the substance appears to reside in the carbohydrate portion of the molecule and certain sugars have been shown to be of critical importance in the specificity of the four blood-group substances studied.

These blood-group substances appear in the human body in two forms. Those in the plasma and secretions are water-soluble whereas those on the cells are ethanol soluble. Attempts are being made to discover whether the latter form can be found on cells other than red cells. As far as blood cells are concerned it seems clear that the A and B antigens are demonstrable on leucocytes and platelets, but the Rh antigens have not been so clearly demonstrated ; a claim to have detected the D antigen on leucocytes and platelets has been advanced, but it has not so far been supported by the use of alternative techniques. It is possible that P is present on leucocytes and platelets (but not on tissue cells) but the Lutheran and Lewis antigens have not been found. If the MN antigens are present on leucocytes and platelets they appear to be in a form rather different from that on the red cells. As far as tissue cells are concerned the A and B substances are certainly present on epidermal cells and on spermatozoa. Traces of the A and B substances have been found in many tissues and relatively high concentrations, particularly in secretors, have been demonstrated in the gastric and duodenal mucosa by means of the fluorescent antibody technique.

In addition to determining the composition of blood group antigens, their situation on the red-cell envelope is also of interest. Each antigen appears to be scattered thinly over the surface disposed in a number of sites. It has been estimated that there are between 2,000 and 5,000 such sites for the Rh antigen D on each red cell ; and many times more for the A antigen. The accessibility of these sites to antibody has never been seriously questioned in human blood groups, but there is evidence in other species that some antigens may not be situated on the outer surface of the cell.

The activity of blood-group antibodies has been the subject of as close an enquiry as has been applied to antigens. The belief that all antibodies are to be found in the *gamma* fraction of serum globulin has recently been called into question. It has been suggested that though most blood-group antibodies are *gamma* globulins some are found among the *alpha* and *beta* fractions of globulin. These latter antibodies seem to unite with the cells only in the presence of complement. There are indications, however, that the supposed non-*gamma* globulin antibodies are, in fact, composed of *gamma* globulin, but that the coincident complement is responsible for the *alpha* or *beta* globulins and is masking the presence of *gamma* globulin on the sensitised cell. There are, nevertheless, two types of blood-group antibody, the form that requires complement for the sensitisation of the cell, and that which does not.

These differences are also reflected in the *in vivo* effects of antibodies on the disposal of cells. Cells sensitised by an incomplete antibody such as anti-D are removed by the spleen with a half-life of some 20 minutes for small experimental samples. Cells sensitised by an antibody that binds complement are removed much more rapidly (half-life about 5 minutes) in the liver. Agglutinating antibodies are also removed by the liver, and hæmolytic antibodies, such as immune anti-A, can bring about intravascular hæmolysis. A physical difference has also been found in comparing naturally-occurring and immune antibodies, the former having a sedimentation constant in the 19S component of *gamma* globulin when studied in the ultra-centrifuge, whereas the latter are found in the 7S component.

A rather unexpected discovery, which is being put to use particularly in chemical studies on blood groups, is that specific agglutinins can be recovered from crushed seeds of certain botanical genera, notably varieties of the Lima bean. Though the term agglutinin is used for these substances they can be thought of, not so much as antibodies but as chemical substances that agglutinate the red cells of certain blood groups. Plant agglutinins with the specificity of anti-A or anti-A_1 have been found, as well as some agglutinating human cells of Groups A, B and AB but not O. Also agglutinins with a specificity of anti-H and anti-N have been discovered.

Genetical studies on human blood have recently extended beyond the confines of the red-blood cells. The antigenic structure of leucocytes also promises to reveal a complexity not far different from that of the erythrocyte. Moreover certain serum globulins have also been shown to be inherited characters. The haptoglobulins, *alpha*-2 globulins capable of binding free hæmoglobin, furnish one example and there are certain *beta* globulins which are also inherited, and the so-called Gm serum groups. These, as well as other interesting and related topics such as the varieties of hæmoglobin and of the sickling gene, are outside the scope of this book.

BIBLIOGRAPHY

It would be impossible to attempt a selection from the mass of papers devoted to one aspect or another of human blood groups. The following monographs, however, will lead the reader to all but the most recent blood group literature.

British Medical Bulletin (1959). *Blood Groups*, Vol. 15.

KABAT, E. A. (1956). *Blood Group Substances, their Chemistry and Immunochemistry.* Academic Press, New York.

MOLLISON, P. L. (1956). *Blood Transfusion in Clinical Practice.* 2nd Ed. Blackwell, Oxford.

MOURANT, A. E. (1954). *The Distribution of Human Blood Groups.* Blackwell, Oxford.

RACE, R. R., and SANGER, RUTH (1958). *Blood Groups in Man.* 3rd Ed. Blackwell, Oxford.

ROBERTS, G. FULTON (1957). *Comparative Aspects of Hæmolytic Disease of the Newborn.* Heinemann, London.

INDEX

Printed in Great Britain
by Amazon

84900480R10051